The Super Easy Bread Cooking Guide

Delicious And Easy Bread Maker Recipes For Everyone

Jude Lamb

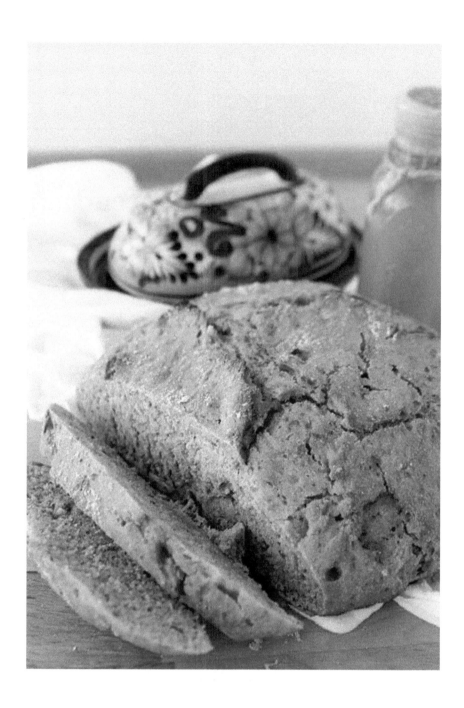

Table of contents

Making Bread...7

Rosemary Garlic Dinner Rolls 9

Egg and Seed Buns 11

Coco-Cilantro Flatbread 13

Parsley Cheddar Bread 15

Lavender Bread...17

Onion Bacon Bread...19

Sunflower & Flax Seed Bread...21

Nutritious 9-Grain Bread 23

Oatmeal Sunflower Bread 25

Cornmeal Whole Wheat Bread 27

Delicious Cranberry Bread 29

Coffee Raisin Bread 31

Healthy Multigrain Bread 33

Italian Pine Nut Bread... 35

Whole Wheat Raisin Bread 37

Healthy Spelt Bread... 39

Sun Vegetable Bread...41

Tomato Onion Bread 43

Tomato Bread... 45

Squash Carrot Bread...47

Curd Onion Bread with Sesame Seeds...50

Banana Bread 52

Blueberry Bread 54

Orange and Walnut Bread 56

Olive Bread with Italian Herbs..59

Banana-Lemon Loaf 61

Australian Vegetable Bread 63

Lemon and Poppy Buns...65

Apple with Pumpkin Bread 67

Peaches and Cream Bread 69

Pure Peach Bread..71

Date Delight Bread..73

Orange Date Bread..75

Zero-Fat Carrot Pineapple Loaf 77

Autumn Treasures Loaf 79

Oatmeal Walnut Bread 81

Pumpkin Raisin Bread...83

Hawaiian Bread...85

Black Forest Loaf 87

Vegan Cinnamon Raisin Bread 89

Beer Bread 91

Onion and Mushroom Bread..93

Low-Carb Multigrain Bread 95

Mashed Potato Bread 97

Honey Sourdough Bread 99

Multigrain Sourdough Bread 101

Sourdough Boule 103

Herbed Baguette 105

Czech Sourdough Bread 107

Sauerkraut Rye..109

Making Bread

There is nothing like the scent of freshly baked bread to greet you when you wake up. Bakers traditionally produced their products during the early hours meaning their loaves were fresh, hot, and mouth-watering tasty for hungry customers wanting a slice of bread to go with a slap-up breakfast.

Bread historically dates back to Neolithic or even prehistoric times in its earliest incarnation.

Prime ingredients include flour and water used to make the dough. The dough can have numerous additives to offer assorted consistency, flavors, and healthy preferences. Additives may include yeast, fat, salt, baking soda, fruits, spices, eggs, milk, sugar, or vegetables. You can even add seeds to the bread, oils, and nuts. Bread is quite a versatile product and can be devoured on its own or as an accompaniment to the main dish. The dough is traditionally baked, but modern alternatives could include steaming.

The outer part of the bread, commonly known as the crust, can be baked into a hard or soft version. The inner part of the bread is classed as the "crumb," strangely not the small bits that cover your lap.

The prime time to eat a loaf of bread is soon after it has been removed from the oven. At this delicious time, the bread is warm, aromatic, and fresh. Leaving the bread for any length of time will cause the bread to become stale.

A quirk dating back to the 13th century was the Baker's Dozen.

A Baker's Dozen, ironic as it was from the 13th century, relates to 13 items making a dozen instead of the usual 1 1/2. As history would have us believe, a Baker's dozen suggested that punishment was administered to bakers who short-changed their customers. One way to ensure that a customer always received a full quota was to give more bread than paid for. Furthermore, if one loaf was damaged, burnt or was of unacceptable quality, there were still 1 1/2 loaves available for the customer.

Another explanation of the Baker's Dozen, and slightly more believable, is that when round loaves were placed on a standard baking tray, the configuration was 3+2+3+2+3 which gave a greater density to the tray and allowed easier stacking.

Over the decades, the baking of bread has followed the path of many traditions updated to reflect the changing needs of society. Whereas bread was always the preserve of the local baker, modern supermarkets now have their own "in-house" ovens, and bread is baked to suit customer demand.

Rosemary Garlic Dinner Rolls

Preparation Time: 20 minutes
1-Pound Loaf

Ingredients:

- ½ teaspoon baking powder
- ½ cup water
- 1/3 cup ground flax seed
- 1 cup mozzarella cheese, shredded
- 1 cup almond flour
- 1 teaspoon rosemary, minced
- A pinch of salt
- 1 oz. cream cheese
- 1 egg, beaten
- 1 tablespoon butter
- 1 teaspoon garlic, minced

Directions:

1. Add all ingredients to the Bread Machine.
2. Select Dough setting. When the time is over, transfer the dough to the floured surface. Shape it into a ball.
3. Roll the dough until it becomes a log and slice into six pounds. Place on a greased baking sheet.

4. Combine rosemary, garlic, and butter in a bowl and mix—brush half of this over the biscuits.

5. Set the heat of the oven to 400° F and bake for 15 minutes.

6. Brush with the remaining mixture and add salt before serving.

Nutrition:

- Calories: 170
- Fat: 19 g
- Carbohydrates: 5.4 g
- Protein: 13 g
- Sodium: 100 mg

Egg and Seed Buns

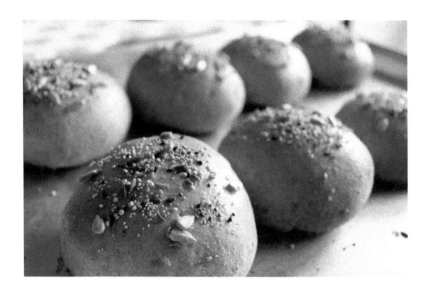

Preparation Time: 15 minutes

1½-Pound Loaf

Ingredients:

- 2 egg whites
- 1 cup sunflower seeds, ground
- ¼ cup flax seeds, ground
- 5 tablespoons psyllium husks
- 1 cup boiling water
- 2 teaspoons baking powder
- Salt to taste

Directions:

1. Combine all the dry ingredients.
2. Add the egg whites and blend until smooth.
3. Add boiling water and keep whisking.
4. Line a baking sheet with parchment paper and drop the dough on it 1 spoonful at a time to form buns.
5. Bake at 356° F for 50 minutes.
6. Serve.

Nutrition:

- Calories: 191
- Fat: 4.2 g
- Carbohydrates: 21 g
- Protein: 3.3 g
- Sodium: 60 mg

Coco-Cilantro Flatbread

Preparation Time: 25 minutes

1-Pound Loaf

Ingredients:

- ☐ ½ cup Coconut Flour
- ☐ 2 tablespoons Flax Meal
- ☐ ¼ teaspoon Baking Soda
- ☐ pinch of Salt
- ☐ 1 tablespoon Coconut Oil
- ☐ 2 tablespoons Chopped Cilantro
- ☐ 1 cup Lukewarm water

Directions:

1. Whisk together the coconut flour, flax, baking soda, and salt in a bowl.
2. Add in the water, coconut oil, and chopped cilantro.
3. Knead it until everything comes together into a smooth dough.
4. Leave to rest for about 15 minutes.
5. Divide the dough into six equal-sized portions.
6. Roll each of it into a ball, then flatten with a rolling pin in between sheets of parchment paper.
7. Refrigerate until ready to use.

8. To cook, heat in a non-stick pan for 2-3 minutes per side.

Nutrition:

- Calories: 176
- Fat: 4 g
- Protein: 1 g
- Carbohydrates: 1 g
- Sodium: 60 mg

Parsley Cheddar Bread

Preparation Time: 15 minutes
2-Pound Loaf

Ingredients:
- 1 tablespoon butter
- 2 tablespoons coconut flour
- 1 large egg
- 1 tablespoon heavy whipping cream
- 2 tablespoons water
- ¼ cup cheddar cheese
- 1 teaspoon garlic powder
- 1 teaspoon onion powder
- 1 teaspoon dried parsley
- 1teaspoon pink Himalayan salt
- 1teaspoon black pepper
- ¼ teaspoon baking powder

Directions:
1. Melt the butter by heating on a coffee mug for 1 second.
2. Slowly stir in seasonings, baking powder, and coconut flour. Mix well using a fork until smooth.
3. Whisk in cream, cheese, water, and egg.

4. Beat well until smooth, then bake for 3 minutes in the microwave.
5. Allow the bread to cool, then serve.

Nutrition:

- Calories: 183
- Total Fat 4 g
- Cholesterol: 27 mg
- Sodium: 39 mg
- Carbohydrates: 9.2 g
- Sugar 3.1 g
- Fiber: 4.6 g
- Protein: 1 g

Lavender Bread

Preparation Time: 20 minutes
1-Pound Loaf

Ingredients:

- ¾ cup lukewarm milk
- 1 tablespoon butter, melted
- 1 tablespoon brown sugar
- ¾ teaspoon salt
- 1 teaspoon fresh lavender flower, chopped
- ¼ teaspoon lemon zest
- ¼ teaspoon fresh thyme, chopped
- 2 cups all-purpose flour, sifted
- ¾ teaspoon active dry yeast

Directions:

1. Prepare all of the ingredients for your bread and measuring means (a cup, a spoon, kitchen scales).
2. Carefully measure the ingredients into the pan.
3. Place all of the ingredients into a bucket in the right order, following the manual for your bread machine.
4. Close the cover.

5. Select the program of your bread machine to BASIC and choose the crust colour to MEDIUM.
6. Press START.
7. Wait until the program completes.
8. When done, take the bucket out and let it cool for 5 minutes.
9. Shake the pound from the pan and let cool for 30 minutes on a cooling rack.
10. Slice, serve, and enjoy the taste of fragrant Homemade Bread.

Nutrition:

- Calories: 163
- Total Fat: 2g
- Saturated Fat: 1g
- Cholesterol: 4g
- Sodium: 221 mg
- Carbohydrates: 25.3g
- Dietary Fiber: 0.9g
- Total Sugars: 1.2g
- Protein: 3.4g
- Vitamin D 1mcg
- Calcium 1 mg
- Potassium 43mg

Onion Bacon Bread

Preparation Time: 1 hour
2-Pound Loaf

Ingredients:

- 1½ cups lukewarm water
- 2 tablespoons sugar
- 3 teaspoons active dry yeast
- 4½ cups wheat flour
- 1 whole egg
- 2 teaspoons kosher salt
- 1 tablespoon olive oil
- 3 small onions, chopped and lightly toasted
- 1 cup bacon, chopped

Directions:

1. Prepare all of the ingredients for your bread and measuring means (a cup, a spoon, kitchen scales).
2. Carefully measure the ingredients into the pan, except the bacon and onion.
3. Place all of the ingredients into a bucket in the right order, following the manual for your bread machine.
4. Close the cover.

5. Select the program of your bread machine to BASIC and choose the crust colour to MEDIUM.
6. Press START.
7. After the machine beeps, add the onion and bacon.
8. Wait until the program completes.
9. When done, take the bucket out and let it cool for 5minutes.
10. Shake the pound from the pan and let cool for 30 minutes on a cooling rack.
11. Slice, serve, and enjoy the taste of fragrant Homemade Bread.

Nutrition:

- Calories: 391
- Fat: 9.7 g
- Cholesterol: 31 g
- Sodium: 480 mg
- Carbohydrates: 59.9 g
- Fiber: 2.1 g

Sunflower & Flax Seed Bread

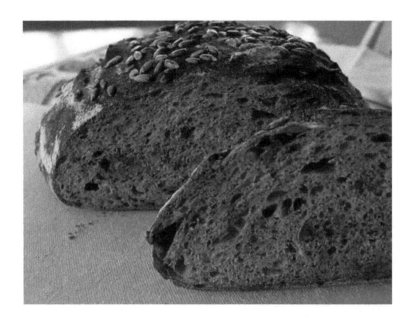

Preparation Time: 30 minutes

2-Pound Loaf

Ingredients:

- 11/3 cups water
- 2 tablespoons butter
- 3 tablespoons honey
- 1½ cups bread flour
- 11/3 cups whole wheat flour
- 1 teaspoon salt
- 1 teaspoon active dry yeast

- ½ cup flax seed
- ½ cup sunflower seeds

Directions:

1. Add all ingredients except for sunflower seeds into the bread machine pan.
2. Select basic setting then select light/medium crust and press start.
3. Add sunflower seeds just before the final kneading cycle.
4. Once pound is done, remove the pound pan from the machine. Allow it to cool for 5 minutes. Slice and serve.

Nutrition:

- Calories: 210
- Carbohydrates: 36.6g
- Fat: 5.7g
- Protein: 6.6g
- Sodium: 240mg

Nutritious 9-Grain Bread

Preparation Time: 10 minutes
1-Pound Loaf

Ingredients:

- ¾ cup+2 tablespoons warm water
- 1 cup whole wheat flour
- 1 cup bread flour
- 9½ cups, crushed 9-grain cereal
- 1 teaspoon salt
- 1 tablespoon butter
- 2 tablespoons sugar
- 1 tablespoon milk powder
- 2 teaspoons active dry yeast

Directions:

1. Put all ingredients into the bread machine.
2. Select whole wheat setting then select light/medium crust and start.
3. Once pound is done, remove the pound pan from the machine.
4. Allow it to cool for 5 minutes. Slice and serve.

Nutrition:

- Calories: 162
- Carbohydrates: 25g
- Fat: 1.7g
- Protein: 4.1g
- Sodium: 160 mg

Oatmeal Sunflower Bread

Preparation Time: 25 minutes
1½-Pound Loaf

Ingredients:

- 1 cup water
- ¼ cup honey
- 2 tablespoons softened butter
- 3 cups bread flour
- ½ cup old fashioned oats
- 2 tablespoons milk powder
- 1 ¼ teaspoons salt
- 2 ¼ teaspoons active dry yeast
- ½ cup sunflower seeds

Directions:

1. Add all ingredients except for sunflower seeds into the bread machine pan.
2. Select basic setting then select light/medium crust and press start. Add sunflower seeds just before the final kneading cycle.
3. Once pound is done, remove the pound pan from the machine. Allow it to cool for 5 minutes. Slice and serve.

Nutrition:

- Calories: 215
- Carbohydrates: 39g
- Fat: 4.2g
- Protein: 5.4g
- Sodium: 300 mg

Cornmeal Whole Wheat Bread

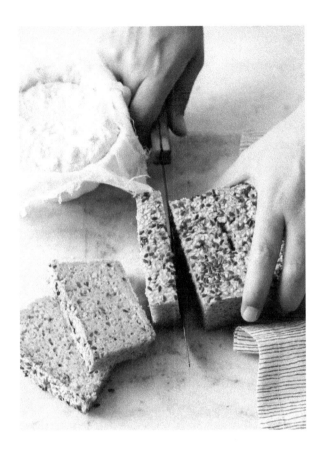

Preparation Time: 10 minutes

2-Pound Loaf

Ingredients:

- 2½ teaspoons active dry yeast
- 1 1/3 cups water
- 2 tablespoons sugar

- 1 egg, lightly beaten
- 2 tablespoons butter
- 1 ½ teaspoons salt
- ¾cup cornmeal
- ¾cup whole wheat flour
- 2¾cups bread flour

Directions:

1. Add all ingredients to the bread machine pan according to the bread machine manufacturer instructions.
2. Select basic bread setting then select medium crust and start. Once pound is done, remove the pound pan from the machine.
3. Allow it to cool for 5 minutes. Slice and serve.

Nutrition:

- Calories: 221
- Carbohydrates: 41 g
- Fat: 3.3 g
- Protein: 7.1 g
- Sodium: 240 mg

Delicious Cranberry Bread

Preparation Time: 10 minutes
2 Pound Loaf

- **Ingredients:**
- 1½ cups warm water
- 2 tablespoons brown sugar
- 1½ teaspoons salt
- 2 tablespoons olive oil
- 4 cups flour
- 1½ teaspoons cinnamon
- 1½ teaspoons cardamom
- 1 cup dried cranberries
- 2 teaspoons yeast

Directions:
1. Put all ingredients to the bread machine in the listed order.
2. Select sweet bread setting then select light/medium crust and start. Once pound is done, remove the pound pan from the machine.
3. Allow it to cool for 1 minute.
4. Slice and serve.

Nutrition:

- Calories: 223
- Carbohydrates: 41.9 g
- Fat: 3.3g
- Protein: 5.5g
- Sodium: 320 mg

Coffee Raisin Bread

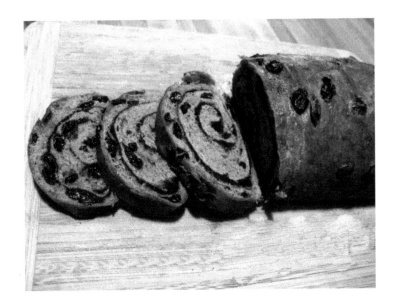

Preparation Time: 10 minutes

2-Pound Loaf

Ingredients:

- 2½ teaspoons active dry yeast
- ¼ teaspoon ground cloves
- ¼ teaspoon ground allspice
- 1 teaspoon ground cinnamon
- 3 tablespoons sugar
- 1 egg, lightly beaten
- 3 tablespoons olive oil
- 1 cup strong brewed coffee

- 3 cups bread flour
- ¾ cup raisins
- 1½ teaspoons salt

Directions:

1. Add all ingredients except for raisins into the bread machine pan.
2. Select basic setting then select light/medium crust and press start. Add raisins just before the final kneading cycle. Once pound is done, remove the pound pan from the machine. Allow it to cool for 5 minutes. Slice and serve.

Nutrition:

- Calories: 230
- Carbohydrates: 41.5 g
- Fat: 5.1 g
- Protein: 5.2 g
- Sodium: 40 mg

Healthy Multigrain Bread

Preparation Time: 10 minutes
1 ½-Pound Loaf

Ingredients:

- 1¼ cups water
- 2 tablespoons butter
- 1 1/3 cups bread flour
- 1½ cups whole wheat flour
- 1 cup multigrain cereal
- 3 tablespoons brown sugar
- 1¼ teaspoons salt
- 2½ teaspoons yeast

Directions:

1. Put ingredients listed into the bread machine pan. Select basic bread setting then select light/medium crust and start.
2. Once pound is done, remove the pound pan from the machine. Allow it to cool for 5 minutes. Slice and serve.

Nutrition:

- Calories: 169
- Carbohydrates: 29.3 g

- Fat: 2.9 g
- Protein: 4.6 g
- Sodium: 260 mg

Italian Pine Nut Bread

Preparation Time: 10 minutes

2-Pound Loaf

Ingredients:

- 1 cup+ 2 tablespoons water
- 3 cups bread flour
- 2 tablespoons sugar
- 1 teaspoon salt
- 5 teaspoons active dry yeast
- 1/3 cup basil pesto
- 2 tablespoons flour
- 1/3 cup pine nuts

Directions:

1. In a small container, combine basil pesto and flour and mix until well blended. Add pine nuts and stir well. Add water, bread flour, sugar, salt, and yeast into the bread machine pan.
2. Select basic setting then select medium crust and press start. Add basil pesto mixture just before the final kneading cycle.
3. Once pound is done, remove the pound pan from the machine. Allow it to cool for 5minutes. Slice and serve.

Nutrition:

- Calories: 210
- Carbohydrates: 34 g
- 32.4g
- Fat: 3.5g
- Protein: 4.1 g
- Sodium: 240 mg

Whole Wheat Raisin Bread

Preparation Time: 25 minutes

1½-Pound Loaf

Ingredients:

- 3½ cups whole wheat flour
- 2 teaspoons dry yeast
- 2 eggs, lightly beaten
- ¼ cup butter, softened
- ¾ cup water
- 1/3 cup milk
- 1 teaspoon salt
- 1/3 cup sugar
- 4 teaspoons cinnamon
- 1 cup raisins

Directions:

1. Add water, milk, butter, and eggs to the bread pan. Add remaining ingredients except for yeast to the bread pan. Make a small hole into the flour with your finger and add yeast to the hole. Make sure yeast will not be mixed with any liquids.

2. Select whole wheat setting then select light/medium crust and start. Once pound is done, remove the pound pan from the machine.
3. Allow it to cool for 5 minutes. Slice and serve.

Nutrition:

- Calories: 290
- Carbohydrates: 53 g
- Fat: 6.2g
- Protein: 6.1 g
- Sodium: 240 mg

Healthy Spelt Bread

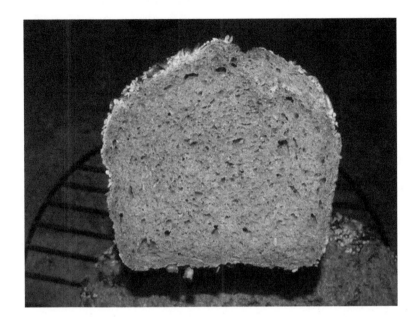

Preparation Time: 10 minutes

1½-Pound Loaf

Ingredients:

- 1¼ cups milk
- 2 tablespoons sugar
- 2 tablespoons olive oil
- 1 teaspoon salt
- 4 cups spelt flour
- 2½ teaspoons yeast

Directions:

1. Add all ingredients according to the bread machine manufacturer's instructions into the bread machine.
2. Select basic bread setting then select light/medium crust and start. Once pound is done, remove the pound pan from the machine.
3. Allow it to cool for 5 minutes. Slice and serve.

Nutrition:

- Calories: 223
- Carbohydrates: 40.3 g
- Fat: 4.5 g
- Protein: 9.2 g
- Sodium: 240 mg

Sun Vegetable Bread

Preparation Time: 10 minutes
1½-Pound Loaf

Ingredients:

- 2 cups (250 g) wheat flour
- 2 cups (250 g) whole-wheat flour
- 2 teaspoons panifarin
- 2 teaspoons yeast
- 1½ teaspoons salt
- 1 tablespoon sugar
- 1 tablespoon paprika dried pounds
- 2 tablespoons dried beets
- 1 tablespoon dried garlic
- 1½ cups water
- 1 tablespoon vegetable oil

Directions:

1. Set baking program, which should be 4 hours; crust color is Medium.
2. Be sure to look at the kneading phase of the dough, to get a smooth and soft bun.

Nutrition:

- Calories: 253
- Total Fat: 2.6 g
- Saturated Fat: 0.5 g
- Cholesterol: 0 g
- Sodium: 444 mg
- Carbohydrate: 49.6 g
- Dietary Fiber: 2.6 g
- Sugars: 0.6 g
- Protein: 7.2 g

Tomato Onion Bread

Preparation Time: 15 minutes
1-Pound Loaf

- **Ingredients:**
- 2 cups all-purpose flour
- 1 cup whole meal flour
- ½ cup warm water
- 2 tablespoons milk
- 3 tablespoons olive oil
- 2 tablespoons sugar
- 1 teaspoon salt
- 2 teaspoons dry yeast
- ½ teaspoon baking powder
- 5 sun-dried tomatoes
- 1 onion
- ¼ teaspoon black pepper

Directions:

1. Prepare all the necessary products. Finely chop the onion and sauté in a frying pan. Cut up the sun-dried tomatoes (5 halves).

2. Pour all liquid ingredients into the bowl; then cover with flour and put in the tomatoes and onions. Pour in the yeast and baking powder, without touching the liquid.
3. Select the baking mode and start. You can choose the Bread with Additives program, and then the bread maker will knead the dough at low speeds.

Nutrition:

- Calories: 241
- Total Fat: 6.4 g
- Saturated Fat: 1.1 g
- Cholesterol: 1 g
- Sodium: 305 mg
- Carbohydrates: 40 g
- Dietary Fiber: 3.5 g
- Sugars: 6.1 g
- Protein: 6 g

Tomato Bread

Preparation Time: 30 minutes
1½ Pound Loaf

Ingredients:

- 3 tablespoons tomato paste
- 1½ cups (340 ml) water
- 4 1/3 cups (560 g) flour
- 1½ tablespoons vegetable oil
- 2 teaspoons sugar
- 2 teaspoons salt
- 1½ teaspoons dry yeast
- ½ teaspoon oregano, dried
- ½ teaspoon ground sweet paprika

Directions:

1. Dilute the tomato paste in warm water. If you do not like the tomato flavor, reduce the amount of tomato paste, but putting less than 1 tablespoon does not make sense, because the color will fade.
2. Prepare the spices. I added a little more oregano as well as Provencal herbs to the oregano and paprika (this bread also begs for spices).

3. Sieve the flour to enrich it with oxygen. Add the spices to the flour and mix well.
4. Pour the vegetable oil into the bread maker container. Add the tomato/water mixture, sugar, salt, and then the flour with spices, and then the yeast.
5. Turn on the bread maker (the Basic program—I have the WHITE BREAD—the crust Medium).
6. After the end of the baking cycle, turn off the bread maker. Remove the bread container and take out the hot bread. Place it on the grate for cooling for 1 hour.

Nutrition:

- Calories: 221
- Total Fat: 3.3 g
- Saturated Fat: 0.6 g
- Cholesterol: 0 g
- Sodium: 440 mg
- Carbohydrate: 54.3 g
- Dietary Fiber: 2.4 g
- Sugars: 1.9 g
- Protein: 7.6 g

Squash Carrot Bread

Preparation Time: 1 hour
1½ Pound Loaf

Ingredients:

- 1 small zucchini
- 1 baby carrot
- 1 cup whey
- 1 ½ cups (11g) white wheat flour
- ¾ cup (10 g) whole wheat flour
- ¾ cup (10 g) rye flour
- 2 tablespoons vegetable oil
- 1 teaspoon yeast, fresh
- 1 teaspoon salt
- ½ teaspoon sugar

Directions:

1. Cut/dice carrots and zucchini to about 15 mm (1/2 inch) in size.
2. In a frying pan, warm the vegetable oil and fry the vegetables over medium heat until soft. If desired, season the vegetables with salt and pepper.

3. Transfer the vegetables to a flat plate so that they cool down more quickly. While still hot, they cannot be added to the dough.
4. Now dissolve the yeast in the serum.
5. Send all kinds of flour, serum with yeast, as well as salt, and sugar to the bakery.
6. Knead the dough in the Dough for the Rolls program.
7. At the very end of the batch, add the vegetables to the dough.
8. After adding vegetables, the dough will become moister. After the fermentation process, which will last about an hour before the doubling of the volume of the dough, shift it onto a thickly floured surface.
9. Turn into a pound and put it in an oiled form.
10. Conceal the form using a food film and leave for 1 to 1 1/3 hours.
11. Preheat oven to 450° F and put bread in it.
12. Bake the bread for 15 minutes, and then gently remove it from the mold. Lay it on the grate and bake for 15 minutes more

Nutrition:

- Calories: 210
- Total Fat: 4.3 g
- Saturated Fat: 0.1 ½ g

- Cholesterol: 0 g
- Sodium: 313 mg
- Carbohydrates: 39.1 g
- Dietary Fiber: 4.1 g
- Total Sugars: 2.7 g
- Protein: 6.6 g

Curd Onion Bread with Sesame Seeds

Preparation Time: 10 minutes
1½-Pound Loaf

Ingredients:

- ¾ cup water
- 32/3cups wheat flour
- 3/4 cup cottage cheese
- 2 tablespoons softened butter
- 2 tablespoons sugar
- 1½ teaspoons salt
- 1½ tablespoons sesame seeds
- 2 tablespoons dried onions
- 1¼ teaspoons dry yeast

Directions:

1. Put the products in the bread maker according to its instructions. I have this order, presented with the ingredients.
2. Bake on the BASIC program.

Nutrition:

- Calories: 277
- Total Fat: 4.7 g

- Saturated Fat: 2.3 g
- Cholesterol: 9 g
- Sodium: 347mg
- Dietary Fiber: 1.9 g
- Sugars: 3.3 g
- Protein: 9.4 g
- Carbohydrates: 41 g

Banana Bread

Preparation Time: 1 hour

1-Pound Loaf

Ingredients:

- 1 teaspoon baking powder
- 1 cup water
- ½ teaspoon baking soda
- 2 bananas, peeled and halved lengthwise
- 2 cups all-purpose flour
- 2 eggs
- 3 tablespoons vegetable oil
- ¾ cup white sugar

Directions:

1. Put Ingredients in the bread pan. Select dough setting. Start and mix for about 3-5 minutes.
2. After 3-5 minutes, press stop. Do not continue to mix. Smooth out the top of the dough.
3. Using the spatula and then select bake, start and bake for about 50 minutes. After 50 minutes, insert a toothpick into the top center to test doneness.

4. Test the pound again. When the bread is completely baked, remove the pan from the machine and let the bread remain in the pan for5minutes. Remove bread and cool in wire rack.

Nutrition:

- Calories: 350
- Carbohydrate: 40 g
- Fat: 13 g
- Protein: 3g

Blueberry Bread

Preparation Time: 1 hour

2-Pounds Loaf

Ingredients:

- 1¼ cups water
- 6 ounces cream cheese, softened
- 2 tablespoons butter or margarine
- ¼ cup sugar
- 2 teaspoons salt
- 4½ cups bread flour
- 1½ teaspoons grated lemon peel
- 2 teaspoons cardamom
- 2 tablespoons nonfat dry milk
- 2½ teaspoons Red Star brand active dry yeast
- 2/3 cup dried blueberries

Directions:

1. Place all ingredients except dried blueberries in the bread pan, using the least amount of liquid listed in the recipe. Select light crust setting and the raisin/nut cycle. Press the start button.

2. Watch the dough as you knead. After 5 minutes, if it is dry and hard or if the machine seems to strain to knead it, add more liquid 1 tablespoon at a time until the dough forms a ball that is soft, tender, and slightly sticky to the touch.
3. When stimulated, add dried cranberries.
4. After the bake cycle is complete, remove the bread from the pan, place it on the cake, and allow it to cool.

Nutrition:
- Calories: 311
- Carbohydrate: 250 g
- Fat: 3 g
- Protein: 9 g
- Sodium: 480 mg

Orange and Walnut Bread

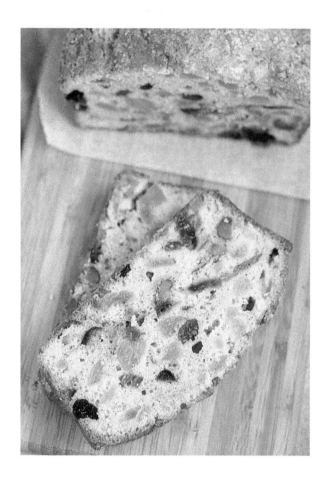

Preparation Time: 1 hour

1-Pound Loaf

Ingredients:

- 1 egg white
- 1 tablespoon water

- ½ cup warm whey
- 1 tablespoon yeast
- 4 tablespoons sugar
- 2 oranges, crushed
- 4 cups flour
- 1 teaspoon salt
- 3 teaspoons orange peel
- 1/3 teaspoon vanilla
- 3 tablespoons walnut and almonds, crushed
- Crushed pepper, salt, cheese for garnish

Directions:
1. Add all of the ingredients to your Bread Machine (except egg white, 1 tablespoon water, and crushed pepper/cheese).
2. Set the program to "Dough" cycle and let the cycle run.
3. Remove the dough (using lightly floured hands) and carefully place it on a floured surface.
4. Cover with a light film/cling paper and let the dough rise for 5minutes.
5. Divide the dough into thirds after it has risen.
6. Place on a lightly flour surface, roll each portion into 1x5 inch sized rectangles

7. Use a sharp knife to cut carefully cut the dough into strips of ½ inch width
8. Pick 2-3 strips and twist them multiple times, making sure to press the ends together
9. Preheat your oven to 400 degrees F
10. Take a bowl and stir egg white, water, and brush onto the breadsticks
11. Sprinkle salt, pepper/ cheese
12. Bake for 15 minutes until golden brown
13. Remove from baking sheet and transfer to cooling rack Serve and enjoy!

Nutrition:

- Calories: 337
- Carbohydrates: 22 g
- Total Fat: 7 g
- Protein: 1½ g
- Sugar: 34 g
- Fiber: 1 g
- Sodium: 240 mg

Olive Bread with Italian Herbs

Preparation Time: 1 hour

1½ -Pound Loaf

Ingredients:

- 1 cup (250 ml) water
- ½ cup brine from olives
- 4 tablespoons butter
- 3 tablespoons sugar
- 2 teaspoons salt
- 4 cups flour
- 2 teaspoons dry yeast
- ½ cup olives
- 1 teaspoon Italian herbs

Directions:

1. Add all liquid products. Then add the butter.
2. Fill with brine and water.
3. Add salt and sugar. Gently pour in the flour and pour the dry yeast in the corners on top of the flour.
4. Send the form to the bread maker and wait for the signal before the last dough kneading to add the olives and herbs.

5. In the meantime, cut olives into 2-3 parts. After the bread maker signals, add it and the Italian herbs into the dough.
6. Then wait again for the bread maker to signal that the bread is ready.
7. Cooled Bread has an exciting structure, not to mention the smell and taste. Bon Appetit!

Nutrition:
- Calories: 272
- Fat: 7.5 g
- Cholesterol: 15 g
- Sodium: 80 mg
- Carbohydrates: 45 g
- Fiber: 3 g

Banana-Lemon Loaf

Preparation Time: 15 minutes
1-Pound Loaf

Ingredients:

- 2 cups all-purpose flour
- ½ cup water
- 1 cup bananas, very ripe and mashed
- 1 cup walnuts, chopped
- 1 cup of sugar
- 1 tablespoon baking powder
- 1 teaspoon lemon peel, grated
- ½ teaspoon salt
- 2 eggs
- ½ cup of vegetable oil
- 2 tablespoons lemon juice

Directions:

1. Put all ingredients into a pan in this order: bananas, wet ingredients, and then dry ingredients.
2. Press the "Quick" or "Cake" setting of your bread machine.
3. Allow the cycles to be completed.

4. Take out the pan from the machine. Then, let cool for5minutes before slicing the bread enjoy.

Nutrition:

- Calories: 311
- Carbohydrates: 15 g
- Fat: 6 g
- Protein: 2 g
- Sodium: 80 mg

Australian Vegetable Bread

Preparation Time: 1 hour

1½-Pound Loaf

Ingredients:

- 4 cups all-purpose flour
- 4 tablespoons sugar
- 2 teaspoons salt
- 2 tablespoons olive oil
- 1 teaspoon yeast
- liquid (3 parts juice + 1-part water)

Directions:

1. Knead in the bread maker four types of dough (3 species with different colours with juice and one kind with water). Take juices of mixed vegetables for coloured liquid:

   > for Bordeaux—juice of beet
   > for red colour—tomato juice
   > for green colour—juice or puree of spinach
   > for white dough—water.

2. While the following kind of dough is kneaded, the previous lump stands warm to raise.
3. Use the Pasta Dough program on your bread maker.

4. The finished white dough was rolled into a large cake, the colour dough of each kind was divided into four pieces each. In a white cake, lay the coloured scones: roll them into small rolls and wrap them in 3 layers in a different order—you get four rolls. Then completely cover the coloured cakes with white dough, create the desired form for the bucket, put it in the bread machine.

5. The program BAKING set the time to 60 minutes. The focus was that the pound resembles plain white bread (as if bread with a surprise)

6. However, the coloured dough was foolish, and sometimes decided to get out.

Nutrition:

- Calories: 225
- Total Fat: 3.3 g
- Saturated Fat: 0.5 g
- Cholesterol: 0 g
- Sodium: 366 mg
- Carbohydrates: 43.1 g
- Dietary Fiber: 1.4 g
- Sugars: 4.9 g
- Protein: 5.3 g

Lemon and Poppy Buns

Preparation Time: 1 hour

1½-Pound Loaf

Ingredients:

- Melted Butter for grease
- 1 1/3 cups hot water
- 3 tablespoons powdered milk
- 2 tablespoons Crisco shortening
- 1½ teaspoon salt
- 1 tablespoon lemon juice
- 4¼ cups bread flour
- ½ teaspoon nutmeg
- 2 teaspoons grated lemon rind
- 2 tablespoons poppy seeds
- 1¼ teaspoons yeast
- 2 teaspoons wheat gluten

Directions:

1. Add all of the ingredients to your Bread Machine (except melted butter).
2. Set the program to "Dough" cycle and let the cycle run.

3. Remove the dough (using lightly floured hands) and carefully place it on a floured surface.
4. Cover with a light film/cling paper and let the dough rise for 5 minutes.
5. Take a large cookie sheet and grease it with butter.
6. Cut the risen dough into 15 pieces and shape them into balls.
7. Place the balls onto the sheet (2 inches apart) and cover.
8. Place in a warm place and let them rise for 30-40 minutes until the dough doubles.
9. Heat your oven to 375 degrees F, transfer the cookie sheet to your oven and bake for 1 ½ -15 minutes. Brush the top with a bit of butter, enjoy!

Nutrition:

- Calories: 231
- Carbohydrates: 31 g
- Total Fat: 11 g
- Protein: 4 g
- Sugar: 1½ g
- Fiber: 1 g
- Sodium: 240 mg

Apple with Pumpkin Bread

Preparation Time: 2 hours 50 minutes
2-Pound Loaf

Ingredients:

- 1/3 cup dried apples, chopped
- 1½ teaspoons bread machine yeast
- 4 cups bread flour
- 1/3 cup ground pecans
- ¼ teaspoon ground nutmeg
- ¼ teaspoon ground ginger
- ¼ teaspoon allspice
- ½ teaspoon ground cinnamon
- 3 teaspoons salt
- 2 tablespoons unsalted butter, cubed
- 1/3 cup dry skim milk powder
- ¼ cup honey
- 2 large eggs, at room temperature
- 2/3 cup pumpkin puree
- 2/3 cup water

Directions:

1. Put all ingredients, except the dried apples, in the bread pan in this order: water, pumpkin puree, eggs, honey, skim milk, butter, salt, allspice, cinnamon, pecans, nutmeg ginger, flour, and yeast.
2. Secure the pan in the machine and lock the lid.
3. Place the dried apples in the fruit and nut dispenser.
4. Turn on the machine. Choose the sweet setting and your desired colour of the crust.
5. Carefully unmold the baked bread once done and allow it to cool for 5 minutes before slicing.

Nutrition:

- Calories: 321
- Carbohydrates: 30 g
- Total Fat: 4 g
- Protein: 11 g
- Sodium: 720 mg

Peaches and Cream Bread

Preparation Time: 10 minutes

1 ½-Pound Loaf

Ingredients:

- ½ cup canned peaches, drained and chopped
- ¼ cup heavy whipping cream, at 80°F
- 1 egg, at room temperature
- ¾ tablespoon melted butter cooled
- 1½ tablespoons sugar
- ¾ teaspoon salt
- ¼ teaspoon ground cinnamon
- 1 ½ teaspoon ground nutmeg
- ¼ cup whole-wheat flour
- 1¾ cups white bread flour
- ¾ teaspoons bread machine or instant yeast

Directions:

1. Put all ingredients as recommended by your bread machine manufacturer.
2. Set the machine for Basic White bread, select medium crust, then press Start.

3. When the pound is finished, remove the bucket from the machine.

4. Let it cool for five minutes.

5. Shake the bucket gently to remove the pound, then turn it out onto a rack to cool.

Nutrition:

- Calories: 253
- Carbohydrates: 27 g
- Total Fat: 4 g
- Protein: 5 g
- Sodium: 180 mg
- Fiber: 1 g

Pure Peach Bread

Preparation Time: 2 hours

1½-Pound Loaf

Ingredients:

- ¾ cup peaches, chopped
- 1/3 cup heavy whipping cream
- 1 egg
- 1 tablespoon butter, melted at room temperature
- 1/3 teaspoon ground cinnamon
- 1½teaspoons ground nutmeg
- 2¼ tablespoons sugar
- 1½ teaspoons salt
- 1/3 cup whole-wheat flour
- 2 2/3 cups white bread flour
- 1 ½ teaspoons instant or bread machine yeast

Directions:

1. Take 1½ pounds size pound pan and add the liquid ingredients and then add the dry ingredients.
2. Place the pound pan in the machine and close its top lid.

3. For selecting a bread cycle, press "Basic Bread/White Bread/Regular Bread," and for choosing a crust type, press "Light" or "Medium."
4. Start the machine, and it will start preparing the bread.
5. After the bread pound is completed, open the lid and take out the pound pan.
6. Allow the pan to cool down for 1 -15 minutes on a wire rack. Gently shake the pan and remove the bread pound.
7. Make pounds and serve.

Nutrition:

- Calories: 201
- Carbohydrates: 11 g
- Total Fat: 0.3 g
- Protein: 1.1 g
- Fiber: 2 g
- Sodium: 240 mg

Date Delight Bread

Preparation Time: 2 hours

1½-Pound Loaf

Ingredients:

- ¾ cup water, lukewarm
- ½ cup milk, lukewarm
- 2 tablespoons butter, melted at room temperature
- ¼ cup honey
- 3 tablespoons molasses
- 1 tablespoon sugar
- 2¼ cups whole-wheat flour
- 1¼ cups white bread flour
- 2 tablespoons skim milk powder
- 1 teaspoon salt
- 1 tablespoon unsweetened cocoa powder
- 1½ teaspoons instant or bread machine yeast
- ¾ cup chopped dates

Directions:

1. Take 1½ pound size pound pan and add the liquid ingredients and then add the dry ingredients. (Do not add the dates as of now.)

2. Place the pound pan in the machine and close its top lid.

3. Plug the bread machine into the power socket. For selecting a bread cycle, press "Basic Bread/White Bread/Regular Bread" or "Fruit/Nut Bread," and for choosing a crust type, press "Light" or "Medium."

4. Start the machine, and it will start preparing the bread. When the machine beeps or signals, add the dates.

5. After the bread pound is completed, open the lid and take out the pound pan.

6. Allow the pan to cool down for 1 -15 minutes on a wire rack. Gently shake the pan and remove the bread pound.

7. Make pounds and serve.

Nutrition:

- Calories: 210
- Carbohydrates: 52 g
- Fat 5 g
- Sodium: 160 mg

Orange Date Bread

Preparation Time: 10 minutes
1-Pound Loaf

Ingredients:

- 2 cups all-purpose flour
- 1 cup dates, chopped
- ¾ cup of sugar
- ½ cup walnuts, chopped
- 2 tablespoons orange rind, grated
- 1½ teaspoons baking powder
- 1 teaspoon baking soda
- ½ cup of orange juice
- ½ cup of water
- 1 pinch salt
- 1 tablespoon vegetable oil
- 1 teaspoon vanilla extract

Directions:

Put the wet ingredients then the dry ingredients into the bread pan.

Press the "Quick" or "Cake" mode of the bread machine.

Allow all cycles to be finished.

Remove the pan from the machine, but keep the bread in the pan for 5 minutes more.

Take out the bread from the pan, and let it cool down completely before slicing.

Nutrition:

- Calories: 210
- Carbohydrates: 1 g
- Fat: 2 g
- Protein: 1 g
- Sodium: 20 mg

Zero-Fat Carrot Pineapple Loaf

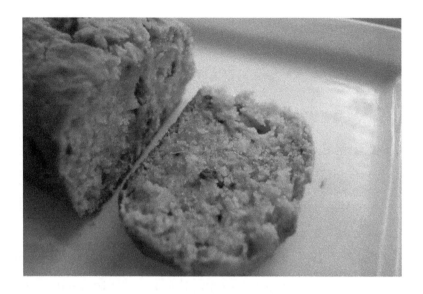

Preparation Time: 10 minutes

1-Pound Loaf

Ingredients:

- 2½ cups all-purpose flour
- ¾ cup of sugar
- ½ cup pineapples, crushed
- ½ cup carrots, grated
- ½ cup raisins
- 2 teaspoons baking powder
- ½ teaspoon ground cinnamon
- ½ teaspoon salt

- ¼ teaspoon allspice
- ¼ teaspoon nutmeg
- ½ cup applesauce
- 1 tablespoon molasses

Directions:
1. Put first the wet ingredients into the bread pan before the dry ingredients.
2. Press the "Quick" or "Cake" mode of your bread machine.
3. Allow the machine to complete all cycles.
4. Take out the pan from the machine, but wait for another 5minutes before transferring the bread into a wire rack.
5. Cool the bread before slicing.

Nutrition:
- Calories: 170
- Carbohydrates: 1 g
- Fat: 0g
- Protein: 1g
- Sodium: 80 mg

Autumn Treasures Loaf

Preparation Time: 15 minutes

1-Pound Loaf

Ingredients:

- 1 cup all-purpose flour
- ½ cup dried fruit, chopped
- ¼ cup pecans, chopped
- ¼ cup of sugar
- 2 tablespoons baking powder
- 1 teaspoon salt
- ¼ teaspoon of baking soda
- ½ teaspoon ground nutmeg
- 1 cup apple juice
- ¼ cup of vegetable oil
- 3 tablespoons aquafaba
- 1 teaspoon of vanilla extract

Directions:

1. Add all wet ingredients first to the bread pan before the dry ingredients.
2. Turn on the bread machine with the "Quick" or "Cake" setting.

3. Wait for all cycles to be finished.
4. Remove the bread pan from the machine.
5. After 5 minutes, transfer the bread from the pan into a wire rack.
6. Slice the bread only when it has completely cooled down.

Nutritions:

- Calories: 210
- Carbohydrates: 1½ g
- Fat: 3g
- Protein: 1 g
- Sodium: 240 mg

Oatmeal Walnut Bread

Preparation Time: 15 minutes

1-Pound Loaf

Ingredients:

- ¾ cup whole-wheat flour
- ¼ cup all-purpose flour
- ½ cup brown sugar
- 1/3 cup walnuts, chopped
- ¼ cup oatmeal
- ¼ teaspoon of baking soda
- 2 tablespoons baking powder
- 1 teaspoon salt
- 1 cup Vegan buttermilk
- ¼ cup of vegetable oil
- 3 tablespoons aquafaba

Directions:

1. Add into the bread pan the wet ingredients then followed by the dry ingredients.
2. Use the "Quick" or "Cake" setting of your bread machine.
3. Allow the cycles to be completed.
4. Take out the pan from the machine.

5. Wait for 5minutes, then remove the bread from the pan.

6. Once the bread has cooled down, slice it and serve.

Nutrition:

- Calories: 220
- Carbohydrates: 11 g
- Fat: 3 g
- Protein: 2 g
- Sodium: 160 mg

Pumpkin Raisin Bread

Preparation Time: 15 minutes
1-Pound Loaf

Ingredients:

- ½ cup all-purpose flour
- ½ cup whole-wheat flour
- ½ cup pumpkin, mashed
- ½ cup raisins
- ¼ cup brown sugar
- 2 tablespoons baking powder
- 1 teaspoon salt
- 1 teaspoon pumpkin pie spice
- ¼ teaspoon baking soda
- ¾ cup apple juice
- ¼ cup of vegetable oil
- 3 tablespoons aquafaba

Directions:

1. Place all ingredients in the bread pan in this order: apple juice, pumpkin, oil, aquafaba, flour, sugar, baking powder, baking soda, salt, pumpkin pie spice, and raisins.
2. Select the "Quick" or "Cake" mode of your bread machine.

3. Let the machine finish all cycles.

4. Remove the pan from the machine. After 5 minutes, transfer the bread to a wire rack.

5. Slice the bread only when it has completely cooled down.

Nutrition:

- Calories: 180
- Carbohydrates: 1½
- Fat: 2 g
- Protein: 1 g
- Sodium: 240 mg

Hawaiian Bread

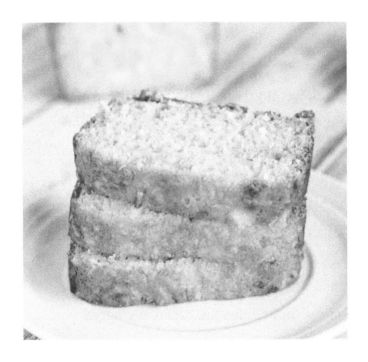

Preparation Time: 10 minutes

1-Pound Loaf

Ingredients:

- 3 cups bread flour
- 2½ tablespoons brown sugar
- ¾ teaspoon salt
- 2 teaspoons quick-rising yeast
- 1 egg
- ¾ cup pineapple juice

- 2 tablespoons almond milk
- 2 tablespoons vegetable oil

Directions:
1. Pour all wet ingredients first into the bread pan before adding the dry ingredients.
2. Set the bread machine to "Basic" or "Normal" mode with a light crust colour setting.
3. Allow the machine to finish the mixing, kneading, and baking cycles.
4. Take out the pan from the machine.
5. Transfer the bread to a wire rack.
6. After one hour, slice the bread and serve.

Nutrition:
- Calories: 190
- Carbohydrates: 30 g
- Fat: 3 g
- Protein: 4 g

Black Forest Loaf

Preparation Time: 1 minute

1 Pound Loaf

Ingredients:

- 1½ cups bread flour
- 1 cup whole wheat flour
- 1 cup rye flour
- 3 tablespoons cocoa
- 1 tablespoon caraway seeds
- 2 teaspoons yeast
- 1½ teaspoons salt
- 1¼ cups water
- 1/3 cup molasses
- 1½ tablespoons canola oil

Directions:

1. Combine the ingredients in the bread pan by putting the wet ingredients first, followed by the dry ones.
2. Press the "Normal" or "Basic" mode and light the bread machine's crust colour setting.
3. After the cycles are completed, take out the bread from the machine.

4. Cool and then slice the bread.

Nutrition:

- Calories: 176
- Carbohydrates: 27 g
- Sodium: 360 mg
- Fat: 2 g
- Protein: 3 g

Vegan Cinnamon Raisin Bread

Preparation Time: 10 minutes
1-Pound Loaf

Ingredients:

- 2¼ cups oat flour
- ¾ cup raisins
- ½ cup almond flour
- ¼ cup of coconut sugar
- 2½ teaspoons cinnamon
- 1 teaspoon baking powder
- ½ teaspoon baking soda
- ¼ teaspoon salt
- ¾ cup of water
- ½ cup of soy milk
- ¼ cup maple syrup
- 3 tablespoons coconut oil
- 1 teaspoon vanilla extract

1. **Directions:**
2. Put all wet ingredients first into the bread pan, followed by the dry ingredients.
3. Set the bread machine to "Quick" or "Cake" mode.

4. Wait until the mixing and baking cycles are done.
5. Remove the pan from the machine.
6. Wait for another 5minutes before transferring the bread to a wire rack.
7. After the bread has completely cooled down, slice it and serve.

Nutrition:
- Calories: 190
- Carbohydrates: 26 g
- Fat: 2 g
- Protein: 3 g
- Sodium: 60 mg

Beer Bread

Preparation Time: 15 minutes

1-Pound Loaf

Ingredients:

- 3 cups bread flour
- 2 tablespoons sugar
- 2¼ teaspoons yeast
- 1½ teaspoons salt
- 2/3 cup beer
- 1/3 cup water
- 2 tablespoons vegetable oil

Directions:

1. Add all ingredients into a pan in this order: water, beer, oil, salt, sugar, flour, and yeast.
2. Start the bread machine with the "Basic" or "Normal" mode on and light to medium crust colour.
3. Let the machine complete all cycles.
4. Take out the pan from the machine.
5. Transfer the beer bread into a wire rack to cool it down for about an hour.
6. Cut into 1½ pounds, and serve.

Nutrition:

- Calories: 180
- Carbohydrates: 25 g
- Fat: 1 g
- Protein: 4 g
- Sodium: 240 mg

Onion and Mushroom Bread

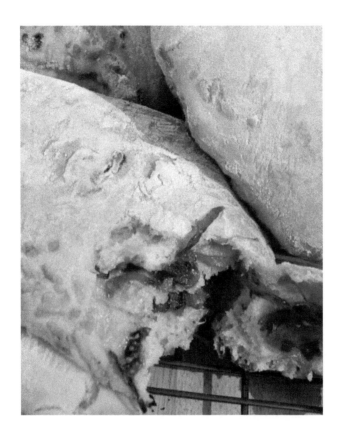

Preparation Time: 10 minutes

1-Pound Loaf

Ingredients:

- 4 ounces mushrooms, chopped
- 4 cups bread flour
- 3 tablespoons sugar

93

- 4 teaspoons fast-acting yeast
- 4 teaspoons dried onions, minced
- 1½ teaspoons salt
- ½ teaspoon garlic powder
- ¾ cup of water

Directions:

1. Pour the water first into the bread pan, and then add all of the dry ingredients.
2. Press the "Fast" cycle mode of the bread machine.
3. Wait until all cycles are completed.
4. Transfer the bread from the pan into a wire rack.
5. Wait for one hour before slicing the bread into 1½ pieces.

Nutrition:

- Calories: 151
- Carbohydrates: 25 g
- Fat: 0 g
- Protein: 5 g

Low-Carb Multigrain Bread

Preparation Time: 15 minutes
1-Pound Loaf

Ingredients:

- ¾ cup whole-wheat flour
- ¼ cup cornmeal
- ¼ cup oatmeal
- 2 tablespoons 7-grain cereals
- 2 tablespoons baking powder
- 1 teaspoon salt
- ¼ teaspoon baking soda
- ¾ cup of water
- ¼ cup of vegetable oil
- ¼ cup of orange juice
- 3 tablespoons aquafaba

Directions:

1. In the bread pan, add the wet ingredients first, then the dry ingredients.
2. Press the "Quick" or "Cake" mode of your bread machine.
3. Wait until all cycles are through.
4. Remove the bread pan from the machine.

5. Let the bread rest for 5 minutes in the pan before taking it out to cool down further.
6. Slice the bread after an hour has passed.

Nutrition:

- Carbohydrates: 9 g
- Fat: 2 g
- Protein: 1 g
- Sodium: 240 mg
- Calories: 175

Mashed Potato Bread

Preparation Time: 40 minutes

1-Pound Loaf

Ingredients:

- 21/3 cups bread flour
- ½ cup mashed potatoes
- 1 tablespoon sugar
- 1 ½ teaspoons yeast
- ¾ teaspoon salt
- ¼ cup potato water
- 1 tablespoon ground flax seeds
- 4 teaspoons oil

Directions:

1. Put the ingredients into the pan in this order: potato water, oil, flax seeds, mashed potatoes, sugar, salt, flour, and yeast.
2. Ready the bread machine by pressing the "Basic" or "Normal" mode with a medium crust colour setting.
3. Allow the bread machine to finish all cycles.
4. Remove the bread pan from the machine.
5. Carefully take the bread from the pan.

6. Put the bread on a wire rack, then cool down before slicing.

Nutrition:

- Calories: 210
- Carbohydrates: 26 g
- Fiber: 2 g
- Sodium: 180 mg

Honey Sourdough Bread

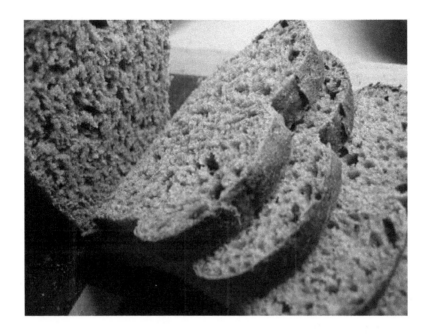

Preparation Time: 15 minutes 1 week (Starter)

1-Pound Loaf

Ingredients:

- 2/3 cup sourdough starter
- ½ cup water
- 1 tablespoon vegetable oil
- 2 tablespoons honey
- ½ teaspoon salt
- ½ cup high Protein: wheat flour
- 2 cups bread flour

- 1 teaspoon active dry yeast

Directions:

1. Measure 1 cup of starter and remaining bread ingredients, add to bread machine pan.
2. Choose basic/white bread cycle with medium or light crust color.

Nutrition:

- Calories: 175
- Carbohydrates: 33 g
- Total Fat: 0.3 g
- Protein: 5.6 g
- Fiber: 1.9 g
- Sodium: 121 mg

Multigrain Sourdough Bread

Preparation Time: 15 minutes; 1 week (Starter)
1-Pound Loaf

Ingredients:

- 2 cups sourdough starter
- 2 tablespoons butter or 2 tablespoons olive oil
- ½ cup milk
- 1 cup water
- 1 teaspoon salt
- ¼ cup honey
- ½ cup sunflower seeds
- ½ cup millet or ½ cup amaranth or ½ cup quinoa
- 3½ cups multi-grain flour

Directions:

1. Add ingredients to bread machine pan.
2. Choose dough cycle.
3. <u>Conventional Oven:</u>
4. When cycle is over, take out dough and place on lightly floured surface and shape into pound.
5. Place in greased pound pan, cover, and rise until bread is a couple inches above the edge.

6. For 40 to 50 minutes, Bake at 375⁰.

Nutrients:

- Calories: 170
- Carbs: 13.5 g
- Total Fat: 1.1 g
- Protein: 2.7 g
- Fiber: 1.4 g
- Sodium: 240 mg

Sourdough Boule

Preparation Time: 4 hours

1 ½-Pound Loaf

Ingredients:

- 1 cup water
- 500 g sourdough starter
- 550 g all-purpose flour
- 1 g salt

Directions:

1. Combine the flour, warm water, and starter, and let sit, covered for at least 30 minutes.
2. After letting it sit, stir in the salt, and turn the dough out onto a floured surface. It should be sticky; you do not have to worry.
3. Flatten the dough slightly (it's best to "slap" it onto the counter), then fold it in half a few times.
4. Cover the dough and let it rise. Repeat the slap and fold a few more times. Now cover the dough and let it rise for 2-4 hours.
5. When the dough at least doubles in size, gently pull it so the top of the dough is taught. Repeat several times. Let it rise for 2-4 hours once more.

6. Preheat to oven to 475° F, and either place a baking stone or a cast iron pan in the oven to preheat.

7. Place the risen dough on the stone or pot, and score the top in several spots. For 1minute, bake then reduce the heat to 425° F, and bake for 25-35 minutes more. The boule will be golden brown.

Nutrition:

- Calories: 243
- Fat: 0.7 g
- Protein: 6.9 g
- Sodium: 10 mg

Herbed Baguette

Preparation Time: 45 minutes

1½-Pound Loaf

Ingredients:

- 5 cups warm water
- 2 cups sourdough starter, either fed or unfed
- 4 to 5 cups all-purpose flour
- 2½ teaspoons salt
- 2 teaspoons sugar
- 1 tablespoon instant yeast
- 1 tablespoon fresh oregano, chopped
- 1 teaspoon fresh rosemary, chopped
- 1 tablespoon fresh basil, chopped
- Any other desired herbs

Directions:

1. In the bowl of a mixer, combine all the ingredients, knead with a dough hook (or use your hands) until a smooth dough is formed—about 7 to 5 minutes, if necessary add more flour.
2. Oil a bowl and place the dough, cover and let it rest for about 2 hours.

3. Beat the dough and divide it into 3 parts. Form each piece of dough into a pound of bread, about 5inches long. You can do this by rolling the dough into a trunk, folding it, rolling it into a trunk, and then folding it again.
4. Place the rolled baguette dough onto lined baking sheets, and cover. Let rise for one hour.
5. Preheat oven to 425F, and bake for 10-25 minutes

Nutrition:
- Calories: 197
- Fat: 0.6 g
- Protein: 5.1 g
- Carbohydrates: 10 g
- Sodium: 400 mg

Czech Sourdough Bread

Preparation Time: 15 minutes; 1 week (Starter)
1-Pound Loaf

Ingredients:

- 1 cup non-dairy milk
- 1 tablespoon salt
- 1 tablespoon honey
- 1 cup sourdough starter
- 1½ cups rye flour
- 1 cup bread flour
- ¾ cup wheat flour
- 1½ cup grated half-baked potato
- 5 tablespoons wheat gluten
- 2 teaspoons caraway seeds

Directions:

1. Add ingredients to bread machine pan.
2. Choose the cycle of dough.
3. The dough should rise, up to 24 hours, in the bread machine until it doubles in size. After rising, bake in the bread machine for one hour.

Nutrition:

- Calories: 191
- Carbohydrates: 39.9 g
- Total Fat: 0.1½ g
- Protein: 6.5 g
- Sodium: 213 mg
- Fiber: 4.3 g

Sauerkraut Rye

Preparation Time: 10 minutes

1-Pound Loaf

Ingredients:

- 1 cup sauerkraut, rinsed and drained
- ¾ cup warm water
- 1½ tablespoons molasses
- 1½ tablespoons butter
- 1½ tablespoons brown sugar
- 1 teaspoon caraway seeds
- 1½ teaspoons salt
- 1 cup rye flour
- 2 cups bread flour
- 1½ teaspoons active dry yeast

Directions:

1. Add all of the ingredients to your bread machine.
2. Set the program of your bread machine to Basic/White Bread and set crust type to Medium
3. Wait until the cycle completes
4. Once the pound is ready, take the bucket out and let the pound cool for 5 minutes

5. Gently shake the bucket to take out the pound.

Nutrition:

- Calories: 174
- Fat: 2 g
- Carbohydrates: 11 g
- Protein: 2 g
- Sodium: 360 mg
- Fiber: 1 g

Lightning Source UK Ltd.
Milton Keynes UK
UKHW020736260521
384399UK00001B/93